The Lord of Birth

The Lord of Birth
Devotional Bible Study for Pregnancy

Birthing Naturally   2005

The Lord of Birth Pregnancy Workbook
© 2005 Jennifer Vanderlaan
www.birthingnaturally.net
All Rights Reserved

Published 2005 by Birthing Naturally, Colonie NY 12205
Printed in the United States of America
ISBN10 0-9765541-0-0
ISBN13 978-0-9765541-0-3

Cover Photo Copyright© Erin Lowery 2003
heart_fullof_faith@yahoo.com

For Josette and Jaron,
whose births taught me more about how to love
and serve God than anything else.

But women will be saved through childbearing –
if they continue in faith, love and holiness with propriety.
1 Timothy 2:15

Contents

Preface

The study you are about to read is a compilation of all the things God taught me about pregnancy, childbirth and myself through my daily times with him during my two pregnancies. Please understand that I am not a biblical scholar, a minister or in any way an authority on the Bible. This work is simply my thoughts and understandings of what I read and how it applied to me.

You may find information in this book that you disagree with. That's ok. The purpose of this book is not to indoctrinate you to my views of Christian childbirth, but to help us all grow closer to God through examining his Word and prayer. Please use the words on these pages in the way that best helps you grow in spiritual maturity.

I hope that God is able to touch your life as much through studying this material as he has touched mine through writing it.

Jennifer Vanderlaan

Chapter One

Does God Care That I Am Pregnant?

Please read 1 Samuel, chapter 1

Perhaps you are a woman like Hannah, who had no doubt that her pregnancy was a gift to her from God. A woman who knew that it was God who caused her to be pregnant and kept her baby safe until it was born. But most likely you are not. The sad truth is that our culture doesn't really think God has anything to do with pregnancy. Sure, we half-heartedly say "Praise God, I'm pregnant," but do we really believe that God had anything to do with it?

We live in the era of do it yourself fertility. When you want your womb closed, you take a pill, use a condom or do anything you can to make sure that sperm and egg don't meet. If they do, we allow women to terminate the pregnancy. When you want the womb opened, you time your sexual encounter to match the latest scientific charts, take a pill, or have a surgery.

Not only do we believe that we make the decisions, we believe our decisions are wise. Perhaps you have always thought you would want to have a child at a certain point in your life, and this is just the natural next step for you. But the standards we use to determine when we should have a child are often the money and convenience, not biblical principles or God's wisdom. Our society does not consider God to be the God of our fertility.

It is not a very far leap from the belief that God had nothing to do with your baby's conception to the belief that God has nothing to do with your pregnancy, and that he probably will be busy on the night you give birth. How sad it would be to travel this exciting time of life without your Lord. How frightening it would be to go through labor without His loving arms supporting you.

The good news is that our society is wrong! God cares very much about your fertility, pregnancy and giving birth. The Bible tells us that God intended children to be a blessing to us, not a curse.

Sons are a heritage from the Lord,
children a reward from him.
Like arrows in the hands of a warrior
are sons born in one's youth.
Blessed is the man whose quiver is full of them.
Psalm 127:3-5a

He will love you and bless you and increase your numbers. He will bless the fruit of your womb, the crops of your land—your grain, new wine and oil— the calves of your herds and the lambs of your flocks in the land that he swore to your forefathers to give you. You will be blessed more than any other people; none of your men or women will be childless, nor any of your livestock without young. Deuteronomy 7:13,14

The Lord will grant you abundant prosperity—in the fruit of your womb, the young of your livestock and the crops of your ground—in the land he swore to your forefathers to give you. Deuteronomy 28:11

Reread those verses again and write down some reasons why God might consider children a blessing.

What is your attitude about children and where do you think it came from?

Based on what you've just read from the Bible, do you need to confess an unbiblical attitude about children? If so, please take a few moments to bring yourself before God. Share with him your hopes, fears, concerns and anything that is on your heart regarding your baby. Write any thoughts here.

If you are still unable or unwilling to accept this pregnancy as part of a blessing from God, stop here and take the time to pray for God to change your heart before you continue this study. Write any thoughts here.

Although our society tells us that we have total control over our bodies, the Bible tells us that the decision if and when to open the womb is always in the hands of God.

> *Then Abraham prayed to God, and God healed Abimelech, his wife and his slave girls so they could have children again, for the Lord had closed up every womb in Abimelech's household because of Abraham's wife Sarah. Genesis: 20:17-18*
>
> *When the Lord saw that Leah was not loved, he opened her womb, but Rachel was barren. Leah became pregnant and gave birth to a son. She named him Reuben, for she said, "It is because the Lord has seen my misery. Surely my husband will love me now." Genesis 29: 31-32*
>
> *Then God remembered Rachel; he listened to her and opened her womb. She became pregnant and gave birth to a son and said, "God has taken away my disgrace." She named him Joseph, and said, "May the Lord add to me another son." Genesis 30:22-24*

But to Hannah he gave a double portion because he loved her, and the Lord had closed her womb. And because the Lord had closed her womb, her rival kept provoking her in order to irritate her. 1 Samuel 1:5-6

In each of these instances, the women wanted to get pregnant. They tried to get pregnant and couldn't. Leah and Rachel were even in a competition to see who could produce the most children, bargaining with each other to sleep with Jacob at certain times.

Without the use of our contemporary fertility drugs and treatments, these women had no choice but to wait for God to determine it was their time to have a baby. They were not a technological society and did not have our understanding of the workings of the human body.

But did they really not have a choice? Every culture has had its doctors, midwives and healers who believed that their treatments and suggestions could encourage fertility. Did they work? Do ours work? Why do we think women today are willing to go through more to get pregnant than women would in biblical times, especially when so much of a woman's value was based on how many children she could produce?

Regardless of technology, God has designed the female body to give cues as to when it is "ripe" for conception. You probably are not aware of these cues unless you have taken a natural family planning class. We have been taught from an early age that the body is mysterious and that only the doctors can understand it. However, the fertility cues still exist. For example, as your body prepares to ovulate, it produces mucus to make the vaginal canal and cervix hospitable to sperm. By paying attention to the difference in mucus that your body produces, you can learn to understand when you are fertile. Leah and Rachel seemed to understand their fertility cues, as they were quick to bargain with each other for the opportunity to sleep with their husband on certain days.

Not only does the Bible tell us that God is in control of our fertility, but it also tells us that God can produce children even without a womb!

And do not think you can say to yourselves, 'We have Abraham as our father.' I tell you that out of these stones God can raise up children for Abraham. Matthew 3:9

Some people try to claim God has nothing to do with conception, that he may have set the system up, but now he just watches from afar. They assume that a loving God would never choose abusive parents or give unwanted children. They wonder why God would open the womb of a young, unmarried woman, for whom the pregnancy will be such a trial.

The problem with this argument is that God never said we should be engaging in fornication. Hebrews 13:4 says "Marriage should be honored by all, and the marriage bed kept pure, for God will judge the adulterer and all the sexually immoral." If we were obedient to God's instruction, unwed pregnancy would not be a problem. God does give us free will, and so does give parents the opportunity to choose selfishness and abuse instead of loving their children.

But if we engage in sin, we can expect some natural consequences. A pregnancy brings the sin into the open and exposes those involved. It also forces those involved to work on difficult issues that arise because of the sin such as broken relationships, selfishness and greed. These problems are not caused by the pregnancy, they are caused by the sin. However, the pregnancy makes it impossible for those involved to ignore the issues any longer. Sometimes, a pregnancy might bring a woman to repentance or draw her closer to God, or it may encourage other women desiring to engage in the same sin to stop pursuing it.

What things make it difficult to believe the Bible when it says it is God who opens the womb?

Who, or what, have you considered besides God to be responsible for your pregnancy?

Since this child, this pregnancy is a blessing from God, he deserves your gratitude. Take a few minutes and write a prayer of thanks to God.

Did you know, not only is your pregnancy a gift from God, but God has also created your child with all her special-ness of personality and character already. God is the creative genius behind genetics, and it is his hand that directs the conception to create just the child he wants. In your body right now dwells a child of God, created for a purpose to meet a need in the Kingdom of God, with all the talents and gifts he will need to fulfill his purpose already! Do you think God cares about your pregnancy? Of course he does!

> *For you created my inmost being;*
> *you knit me together in my mother's womb.*
> *I praise you because I am fearfully and wonderfully made;*
> *your works are wonderful, I know that full well.*
> *Psalm 139:13-14*

> *"Before I made you in your mother's womb, I chose you. Before you were born, I set you apart for a special work. I appointed you as a prophet to the nations." Jeremiah 1:5*

Has what you've learned changed the way you feel about this pregnancy? Has it changed the way you think about your baby? As you end this chapter, take some time to journal your thoughts and feelings about this pregnancy.

A Personal Discipline

This week concentrate on the way you talk about your baby, this pregnancy and the changes you are going through. Do your words recognize your child and this pregnancy as a blessing? Do your words recognize God as the source of this blessing? Do your words convey your thanks for this wonderful gift that God has given you? If not, change your words! Don't allow yourself to speak about this blessing from God as a curse, or to be ungrateful for this gift.

Chapter Two

It's All in the Attitude

Being thankful for the blessing of your baby may not be enough to make you feel comfortable with your pregnancy. Even with overflowing joy, most women still have concerns. Every woman has her own set of doubts when she becomes pregnant. Every woman, no matter how much she has longed for the baby, feels some fear, concern or worry. Each woman's list is unique, reflecting her circumstances.

As you read through the list of possible concerns, consider your own life, your situation, and your heart. Where is your heart today? Where has it been this week? Have you spent time in agony, anger or fear? Have you been anxious, worried or hopeless?

Will the baby be healthy?

Will labor hurt?

Will I have stretch marks?

How will I pay for all the baby equipment?

Will I be a good mother?

Am I eating right?

What if it isn't my doctor on call?

Will the baby's room be ready in time?

Will my water break in the grocery store?

Is it ok to take this cold medicine?

Is it ok not to take these vitamins?

Should I be exercising?

Should I be resting?

Will I have to watch children's programs?

Will I be able to stay home with the baby?

Will I be able to go back to work?

Will my other children accept the new baby?

Does my husband want this baby as much as I do?

What if I don't really want to be pregnant?

When will I feel safe that I won't miscarry?

When will I stop throwing up?

Does my back have to hurt so much?

Does nursing hurt?

What if my husband thinks I am ugly pregnant?

What if I don't want to share my body?

What if my baby comes early?

What if my baby comes late?

Am I eating enough?

Am I eating too much?

Will I be able to lose this weight after the baby?

Will I lose my figure forever?

Am I a bad person for not wanting this baby?

Were any of these your worries? Do you recognize yourself in any of these questions? Read the list again, marking the concerns you feel and adding any you have that are not listed.

Read these verses from Philippians 4:6-7, then rewrite it in your own words to reflect your anxieties about this pregnancy.

> *Do not be anxious about anything, but in everything, by prayer and petition, with thanksgiving, present your requests to God. And the peace of God, which transcends all understanding, will guard your hearts and your minds in Christ Jesus.*

How do these verses make you feel about your list of concerns?

Being honest, take a moment to consider how much time you spend worrying about this pregnancy.

It is a shame that we allow Satan to rob our peace and joy by making us feel "busy" as we focus on everything we think we need to get done. When you are pregnant, your body is working overtime as it tries to feed, breathe for and clean the blood of two individuals, so you start the day more tired than if you were not pregnant. Add to that the hormone changes, not being comfortable as your body readjusts to a new center of gravity and carrying 40 extra pounds and it can be very easy to get overwhelmed with your daily tasks.

But a pregnant woman is not just focused on her daily life, she is also focused on her list of anxieties. Let's be honest here. Of course you do need to think about what you are going to eat, and you need to plan a shopping list and pick up food from the grocery store, but did you go beyond the "preparation" plans? What about concerns of your baby's health or losing your baby? Do you have a concern based on information your caregiver (doctor or midwife) gave you, or based on your own fears?

A good test of your worry is to look at the fruit it brings into your life. Yes, there will be fruit in your life from worry.

> *...they will eat the fruit of their ways*
> *and be filled with the fruit of their schemes. Proverbs 1:31*

> *"Make a tree good and its fruit will be good, or make a tree bad and its fruit will be bad, for a tree is recognized by its fruit. Matthew 12:33*

If it was a healthy, God given concern, such as "I should try getting some exercise a few days a week to keep my strength up," it should have encouraged you to take a specific action. In this case, perhaps a walk around your neighborhood after dinner. This is good fruit. God has made you aware of something you need to do, and you have done it.

If your worry was not healthy, and not a God given concern, there will probably be no specific action you are encouraged to take. Instead, you will find that your time has been wasted, you are more exhausted than when you began to worry, and nothing about the situation has changed. This is bad fruit. Satan has used this to cause you to lose faith in God.

Take a few minutes to write out your worries and the fruit they have produced.

Worry is sinful because it shows a lack of trust in God. It is easy to say you trust God when everything is going well. But the true test of your trust in God is if you trust him when things get difficult. It is only trust when you need to trust.

Because of the "mysterious" nature of pregnancy (not being able to see the baby, but knowing he's there, unsure of when he'll be born, what does he look like, etc) it is a great time to strengthen your trust in God. How do you do that? You can start through prayer and Bible reading!

Read the following verses, and write, in your own words, what each one means to you specifically in this pregnancy.

And we know that in all things God works for the good of those who love him, who have been called according to his purpose. Romans 8:28

Jesus looked at them and said, "With man this is impossible, but not with God; all things are possible with God."
Mark 10:27

Those who know your name will trust in you, for you, Lord, have never forsaken those who seek you. Psalm 9:10

As you end this chapter, simply present your requests to God. Tell him honestly what you are afraid of, even if you think it makes you a bad person. You cannot shock God, he's seen it all. Tell him your concerns; tell him why they concern you. As you pour your heart out to God, don't forget to thank him, and rejoice in him. If you have a worrisome personality, you may not think there is anything to thank God for, but there always is. For every concern you give him, try to find two things to thank God for and rejoice in him.

A Personal Discipline:

For the next week, every time you worry about anything concerning this pregnancy, begin to pray to God, asking him to show you what you need to do or take the worry away. It is ok to ask him to send a clear answer so you will understand. Be sure to write down the answer from God. At the end of the week, look back over your list. Do you see a steady decline in the amount of time you spent worrying? Do you notice any patterns of worry? If there is one topic that continually comes up for worry, spend a good amount of time praying about it.

Chapter Three

Why is Labor so Bad?

I have heard two sides of the issue of pain in labor, both presented with arguments from the Bible to prove that they are legitimate. We are going to take some time to review both of these arguments, and try to determine where the truth lies.

Do you remember reading in Genesis that Eve ate the apple first? Do you remember what God told Eve would happen because she ate that apple? You probably do, because it has become common knowledge that God cursed women to have pain in birth because Eve sinned.

> To the woman he said, "I will greatly increase your pains
> in childbearing; with pain you will give birth to children.
> Your desire will be for your husband, and he will rule over
> you." Genesis 3:16

Some experts on that garden scene will go into great detail about why every woman must have pain in labor to pay for this grave sin, and some go so far as to say that pain medication in labor is an even worse sin because it takes away the woman's punishment.

You can breathe a sigh of relief now, because I am not one of those experts. I have found three real big problems with the belief that labor is supposed to be painful as a curse. First, not all women experience painful births! I am not just talking about the women who use medication to numb the pain. There are women who have natural births (vaginal, without medication) who honestly could not describe the sensations that they felt as "painful." There are even women who describe labor as enjoyable! If this pain of labor was a curse on womanhood, it couldn't skip random women.

The second problem is that God considers children to be a blessing, not a curse. The Bible repeatedly tells us that children are a reward and a blessing to those he loves. I am not suggesting that all blessings will be comfortable and enjoyable all the time, there are very difficult times in raising children. However, a blessing should be a source of Joy. How could a child be, at the same time a blessing and a curse? It simply does not make sense.

> *Sons are a heritage from the Lord,*
> *children a reward from him.*
> *Like arrows in the hands of a warrior*
> *are sons born in one's youth.*
> *Blessed is the man whose quiver is full of them. Psalm 127:3-5*

> *He will love you and bless you and increase your numbers. He will bless the fruit of your womb, the crops of your land—your grain, new wine and oil—the calves of your herds and the lambs of your flocks in the land that he swore to your forefathers to give you. You will be blessed more than any other people; none of your men or women will be childless, nor any of your livestock without young. Deuteronomy 7:13*

> *The Lord will grant you abundant prosperity—in the fruit of your womb, the young of your livestock and the crops of your ground—in the land he swore to your forefathers to give you. Deuteronomy 28:11*

The third reason I do not believe that statement is a curse has to do with the actual meanings of the Hebrew words used. The word that is translated as "to increase" in addition to its meaning of increasing, is also a word that means to be in authority over. The word that is translated as childbearing actually means conception or fertility. So the statement may be of God's authority over fertility.

The words translated as pain in the first and second half of the sentence are different words! In fact, the word used in the first half of the sentence is the exact same word that is translated as toil (hard work) when God spoke to Adam. So, it is possible that the "curse" may mean:

16

"I will have authority over your labor and fertility. With toil (hard work) you will have children."

This understanding makes much more sense to me with the second half of the statement that tells the woman that she will desire her husband, and he will be an authority over her. Perhaps God's famous "curse" is not a curse at all, but a statement of the authority women will now be under.

This also makes sense with the following verses in which Paul states a woman must remain under the authority of the husband.

> *I do not permit a woman to teach or to have authority over a man; she must be silent. For Adam was formed first, then Eve. And Adam was not the one deceived; it was the woman who was deceived and became a sinner. But women will be saved through childbearing – if they continue in faith, love and holiness with propriety.*
> *1 Timothy 2:12-15*

The Genesis and 1 Timothy verses seem to mirror each other. The Genesis verse when paraphrased says, "I am going to be the authority of your fertility. Your husband is going to be the authority over the family." The 1 Timothy verse when paraphrased says, "The husband is the authority of the family, but the woman doesn't have to be overcome by birth if she continues in faith, love and holiness with propriety."

Some teachers have tried to say that the salvation talked about in 1 Timothy is the salvation all mankind received through Christ who was born of a woman. Others believe that this verse means that a woman will become more Christ-like for having gone through birth, therefore being more willing to accept Christ and be saved.

The problem is that these suggestions look at the word saved as if it referred to eternal salvation. However, the Greek word used here for "saved" is a temporal salvation, as if saved from a specific event or time, for example, if you were "saved" from a fire, or "saved" during an accident. When it says a woman can be saved through childbearing, I believe it means she can prevent excessive work during her labor. Simply put, God did not curse women any more than he cursed men.

The other argument about pain in childbirth that I frequently hear is that childbirth should not be painful. Those who believe this theory state that we have been redeemed from the "curse" and that faith in God should be enough to get a woman through labor without pain. I will admit that I tend to fall into this category; however I do not follow it to its extreme. Although I do believe that faith in God can and does help prevent problems in labor that stem from the fear-tension-pain cycle outlined by Dr. Dick-Read, I don't think faith alone can or does prevent all pain.

I have noticed in my reading of the bible that God seems less concerned about the comfort of his people then he is in the character of his people. When Paul complained of a thorn in his side, God did not remove it but rather told him, "My grace is sufficient for you, for my power is made perfect in weakness." 2 Corinthians 12:9. When Lot was urged to leave Sodom, God did not whisk him away, but rather told him to run quickly and not look back. Noah was not given a boat, he was given the plans for a boat that he needed to construct himself. God does provide us with protection, but it can and does frequently require work on our part. It seems natural to me that when it comes to giving birth, God would give us the tools needed to handle it, and allow us to strengthen our faith in him by using those tools.

Think of a difficult time in your life. What tools did God give you to handle the situation? How did that situation impact your relationship with God?

The truth is, there can be many reasons why a labor is painful, and a difficult labor is not necessarily an indication of a lack of faith. There are some ways to ready yourself for the best possible labor, however even these are not a guarantee that you will have the "perfect" labor. It is important to remember that in labor, as in any part of life, you don't always get to choose what happens. God remains in control, and sometimes God's plan is different from your plan. That being said, lets take a look at ways to help prevent unnecessary pain during labor.

*Examine yourselves to see whether you are in the faith;
test yourselves. Do you not realize that Christ Jesus is in
you–unless, of course, you fail the test?
2 Corinthians 13:5*

Although a lack of faith is not the only problem in labor, it can
be a problem in labor. When faith is lacking, fear becomes a
driving force in the body. Fear can do damage to a labor
because the chemicals the body uses to communicate fear will
slow down or even stop the labor process. We will discuss more
about faith in labor in chapter 6, but for now just know you need
to trust God to eliminate fear.

What, if anything, are you fearful of as you advance through this
pregnancy?

Another problem in labor is a lack of obedience to God. Un-
confessed sin separates us from God. We are told that he
"hides" his face from us. You may think that you have been
depending on the strength of God, but if you have unrepentant
sin in your life, you are actually working on your own strength.
God takes sin very seriously, he has to. His Holiness will not
allow him to dwell where there is sin, so unrepentant sin is like
kicking God out of your life. It is vitally important that as
Christians we are in prayer daily, seeking forgiveness for sins.

Spend a few minutes examining your heart. What, if anything, do
you need to confess to God?

Some women suffer through difficult labors because of a lack
of good stewardship. The principle of stewardship is that you are
only a caretaker of the things you possess, that they actually
belong to God. As the caretaker, steward, of Gods things you are
to use your resources wisely, making the most of every
opportunity. Read Matthew 15:14-30 for Jesus' parable about the
talents to understand the concept of stewardship.

Regardless of how many material items or possessions God has or has not entrusted to you, you have been trusted with your body.

> *Do you not know that your body is a temple of the Holy Spirit, who is in you, whom you have received from God? You are not your own; 1 Corinthians 6:19*

As the caretaker of your human body, it is your responsibility to see that your body is properly cared for and maintained in the best possible health. A lack of good nutrition and exercise during pregnancy leaves the body weak and functioning poorly. It also increases your risk for complications during labor. It is also possible to make poor stewardship decisions regarding the amount of stress or work that you make your body do. Some women overwork their bodies; others stop their bodies from any work.

In what ways have you demonstrated good stewardship of your body?

In what ways can you improve your stewardship of your body?

Another spiritual discipline that will help you in labor is to be prepared for what is coming. In the book of Nehemiah we watch as the cupbearer to the king rebuilds the city of Jerusalem. Yet, he does not just show up and start building. Nehemiah seeks the permission of the king and gets his help in making preparations for the project. He has the king write letters to ensure safe passage to Jerusalem, to provide the materials needed for the work, and the king provided army officials to travel with him. Even when he arrived at the city, Nehemiah continued to prepare before he began his work. He surveyed the work to be done before he brought the project to the nobles and priests because he knew he would have opposition and he needed to be prepared for it. When the work did begin, Nehemiah's preparations helped make the rebuilding of the city successful.

It is unfortunate that some women will try to labor without ever having prepared to give birth. They do not take the time to train themselves in labor techniques or practice comfort measures. It is foolish to think that you would be able to use a skill that you have not given yourself the time needed to develop. The more you practice natural childbirth techniques the better they will work for you in labor. This is for two reasons. First, because the more you practice the more familiar you become with what techniques work well for you. Secondly, because the more you practice the better able you are to use the technique during a stressful situation.

In what ways have you already begun to prepare to give birth?

In what ways can you improve your preparation to give birth?

Even with all the right attitudes and with proper preparation it is still possible that your labor may be difficult. We can learn a lesson from Job, a righteous man and praised by God. Yet God still allowed Job to suffer for a time with pain and loss for no apparent reason other than to prove his faithfulness and to bring glory to God. This is very important to remember, because being a Christian and being righteous is not a guarantee of an easy life or an easy labor.

The Bible tells us that God's ways are higher than our ways, and that the wisdom of man is foolishness to God (1 Corinthians 1:25, Isaiah 55:9). We cannot understand why God chooses to give one woman the blessing of an easy labor while another woman labors with difficulty and complication. What we do know is that when tested with adversity, God can give us the strength to persevere. You cannot choose the circumstances of your child's birth, but you can choose how you respond to the circumstances. Although you are not promised an easier labor by relying on God, it is still important to be in a right relationship with him. You cannot draw on God for strength through adversity if you are not in a right relationship with Him.

A Personal Discipline

This week, take some time to review the spiritual disciplines that you need to work on. Make a definite plan about how to improve that discipline over the next few days and then put that plan into action. If necessary, ask a friend or loved on to hold you accountable to your plan.

Chapter Four

Preparation and Training
Following the Example of Mary and Elizabeth

Please read the first chapter of Luke. It is the section where Elizabeth and Mary are told that they will be pregnant. Did you notice what Mary did? Read this section again.

> *At that time Mary got ready and hurried to a town in the hill country of Judea, where she entered Zechariah's home and greeted Elizabeth.*

Mary went to her relative Elizabeth because she knew Elizabeth was pregnant. We are told that Mary was visited by Gabriel while Elizabeth was in her sixth month, and after receiving the message, hurried to be with Elizabeth. We are then told that Mary stayed with her for three months. It is possible that Mary was with Elizabeth during the birth of Elizabeth's son, which we are told about at the end of Chapter one.

Why is it important to know where Mary spent three months of her pregnancy? Because by staying with her relative, Mary was preparing herself for what she would be going through in just a few months. Mary was learning from Elizabeth what she would need to do to stay healthy during pregnancy and how to prepare to give birth. We can consider their relationship during these three months to be a mentoring relationship.

In Titus, the Bible tells us that women should be in mentoring relationships with older, more mature women. This is an excellent way to learn how to be a woman of God.

Likewise, teach the older women to be reverent in the way they live, not to be slanderers or addicted to much wine, but to teach what is good. Then they can train the younger women to love their husbands and children, to be self-controlled and pure, to be busy at home, to be kind, and to be subject to their husbands, so that no one will malign the word of God. Titus 2:3-5

A mentoring relationship works well because you develop a close, trusting relationship with your mentor. You learn not only by her instruction, but also by her example. By watching what she does, and how she handles situations, you will grow yourself. In the relationship, you can ask questions, seek advice and deal with issues that may not be appropriate in a larger group.

The best mentoring relationships do not come from planned "study" groups of women, but from friendships in which women share their complete lives with each other. It happens when they share where they have struggled, how they have grown and what they have learned.

Chances are you have had this type of relationship with one or more women, but had never really thought of it as a mentoring relationship. And you may also have been the one in a relationship who teaches another woman.

Take a few minutes to think who have been your mentors, and what did you learn from them? Then think about who you may have mentored, and what you have taught them. If you have never had a mentoring relationship, take a few minutes to figure out why. Ask God to reveal to you how to take your friendships to a deeper level so you and your women friends can share your hurts, struggles and growth.

Take a minute to reread the Titus 2 verses. Rewrite it in a way that helps you understand its application to pregnancy and giving birth.

A "birth mentor" may be a strange concept to you. Indeed, it does warrant some explanation. In our culture, birth is a very private and hidden event.   But this was not always the case. There is a special connection between women who are pregnant. Have you been in conversation with another pregnant woman yet? Did you ask each other questions about weight gain, back aches and frequent trips to the bathroom? Did you find comfort in knowing you are not the only woman who can't wear her shoes any more? Were you encouraged by your conversation? I hope so.

For thousands of years, women shared their births with other women in the community, their friends and family. The women would assist the mother by helping her stay comfortable and providing the medical help that was available to them.   The mother would assist the women by her example to those who had not yet given birth.   In this system, both the mother and the community women benefited.   This also ensured that each generation of women would be prepared to undergo labor and birth.

When birth was relegated to being a "medical" event, it was moved from the supportive community of women to lonely, sterile hospital wards. Suddenly, women were expected to know how to give birth without ever really understanding what would be happening to their body. Instead of learning the skills necessary to give birth naturally, women were only told stories of the pain they would feel. Birth went from being a normal part of life to a frightening event to be escaped and avoided.

We are very fortunate to have left the "dark ages" of birth behind us.   Hospitals all over our country are now allowing women the freedom they desire for their births. Gone are the days of isolation, we have returned to the days of supporting women as they labor. But we have not returned to the days of training women to give birth by allowing them to learn from other women's births.

If we are to follow the example that Mary and Elizabeth set, we must do two things. First, find a birth mentor. This should be a woman who is further in her pregnancy than you who will include you in her natural childbirth preparation classes and train you to assist her during her labor. Then, when she is in labor, you will do your part to keep her comfortable, relaxed and focusing on the task at hand.

The second thing we must do is to find someone to mentor. This will be a woman who is not as far along as you in her pregnancy, or maybe only planning to become pregnant soon. Perhaps you will have two or three women you mentor. You will include her in your birth preparations, teaching her how to stay comfortable and healthy during pregnancy, and then allowing her to assist you at your birth.

Understand that you are not there just to "watch" or to "witness" your mentor give birth, although you will do that. You will have an active part in her labor, acting as her servant and meeting her needs. The needs will vary with each birth. The woman may wish you to rub her back, or ask you to be sure she drinks water, or may use you as a support as she walks through contractions, or she may ask you to do all three. This is an active relationship that is a partnership through the birth. You are there not only to learn, but also to minister to her needs at that time. When you are in labor, the woman you train will do the same for you.

Take a few moments to think about your strengths and talents, and what you would be comfortable learning. What types of things might you be able to do for a birth mentor?

Take a few moments to think about who you are, what makes you comfortable and relaxed. What types of things might you train a friend to be able to do for you?

The birth student does not take the place of the husband, doctor or midwife, or a professional doula (labor assistant) that you have hired. She will be an "assistant coach," working with the doula and husband to ensure your comfort. She will not be responsible for your medical care like the caregiver, nor will she be required to make decisions for you or your husband. She is there only for emotional support and physical comfort.

It is important that when you select your mentor and your student, that you select women who consider labor and giving birth to be a serious matter. For example, if she is interested but doesn't want you to attend classes, or doesn't want to attend classes with you, you may need to find someone else who is more willing to learn and to teach.

As you end your time with God today, pray that he will give you wisdom in: choosing a birth mentor and a birth student; selecting books about birth to help prepare you; selecting natural birth classes that will help prepare you; and selecting caregivers who will be respectful of your wishes for your birth.

A Personal Discipline:

As you read about the "birth mentor" relationship, did God place the names of any women on your heart? Go to God in prayer right now, asking him to reveal to you who would be best suited to be your birth mentor, and who you should invite as your birth student.

After much prayer, talk the woman you think God is leading you to and discuss with her the birth mentor relationship. If she agrees, humble yourself to the level of her servant, learning from her what you will need to know to serve her at her birth. Once that relationship is established, then pray for and enlist the help of the woman who God is leading you to ask to be your birth student.

Chapter Five

Inviting God to Your Baby's Birth

When you are dealing with morning sickness, weight fluctuations, sleepless nights and frequent bathroom breaks, it is pretty easy to see your pregnant body as "under attack." What may be less obvious is the spiritual battleground that grows with your ever-expanding belly. As you work through the challenges of labor, you will also be working through spiritual challenges.

We live in a society that trusts in its technology. There seems to be a general belief that technology is safer, more accurate and faster, so it is good. Unfortunately, trusting in technology often means that we do not trust in God. We see this in the psalms when we are told:

> *Some trust in chariots and some in horses, but we trust in the name of the Lord our God. Psalm 20:7*

Read the passages surrounding this verse, then re-write its meaning.

In what ways can this verse be related to childbirth?

> *I do not trust in my bow,*
> *my sword does not bring me victory;*
> *but you give us victory over our enemies,*
> *you put our adversaries to shame.*
> *In God we make our boast all day long,*
> *and we will praise your name forever. Psalm 44:6-8*

Technology is a gift from God. We can use computers to keep in touch with friends and relatives who are in other states or other countries. The telephone can bring help in a matter of minutes when you dial 911. Many tools and utensils allow us to get our work done faster and easier. Technology can also save a life when a placenta has prematurely pulled away from the uterine wall. Unfortunately, technology can become like a god for us when we stop thinking of it as a tool available to us, and start believing it is necessary for existence.

> *They exchanged the truth of God for a lie, and worshiped and served created things rather than the Creator—who is forever praised. Amen. Romans 1:25*

When we worship the creation rather then the creator, we make for ourselves an idol. God has commanded us to not serve idols, but to serve and worship only God. He should be our source of comfort; God should be our source of salvation.

> *And God spoke all these words:*
> *"I am the Lord your God, who brought you out of Egypt, out of the land of slavery. You shall have no other gods before me.*
> *You shall not make for yourself an idol in the form of anything in heaven above or on the earth beneath or in the waters below." Exodus 20:1-4*

But we have gone so far as to even make ourselves a new savior, one of flesh and blood who will worship our idols with us. Rather than turn our fears over to God in prayer, we turn them over to caregivers (doctors and midwives) as requests for medication. Rather than allow God to demonstrate his power by delivering us from the pain of birth, we ask the caregiver to deliver us from birth. It is all very subtle, but in our attempt to lessen our pain, we remove the only true source of strength and help. By allowing the caregiver and his medicine to be our god, we kick the Holy God out of the labor and birth room. Yes, God did send us doctors and midwives to help us; God did not send us caregivers to take away the process of giving birth from us.

Labor is a process that God set up because it works. Not only does it work, but each important step in a labor and birth helps to prepare for the next step, and prevent problems. Labor becomes dangerous when we try to prevent certain steps from happening, or hurry to the next step before our bodies are ready.

Some women do experience problems in their births, but this number is somewhere around 5%. The rest of the "problems" experienced in birth may not have been a result of birth at all. Each intervention that is used increases risks for both the mother and the baby. When you are dealing with a normal labor, using medications adds risks that would not have been there. When your goal is a healthy mom and a healthy baby, your decisions need to be made by determining how you keep the level of risk the lowest possible. In most cases, this is without medications.

It takes honesty and wisdom to determine if what you are experiencing is a real problem that needs intervention. I can not even begin to tell you how important it is that you attend a good class in natural childbirth. Your chances of having a normal birth jump significantly when you understand the normal labor process and the effects of the options available. If the class you are taking does not tell you benefits and risks of certain procedures or interventions, then you do not have the information you need to make an informed choice.

Many medical based birth classes are set up to explain to you what the caregiver will do, what is expected of you, and then teach you a few breathing and relaxation exercises. But in many cases these classes are really saying to you "Your body has been created defectively. You couldn't possibly do this on your own, because your body wasn't equipped to handle it. You better let us take care of it or you and your baby will die." These classes teach women that God is powerless to help them through birth.

Have you met people with this attitude yet? Have the women at work, or in the mall, or even at church told you just how terrible labor is and that you better get the drugs because they are the only thing that can help? What are they really saying about God if they believe the drugs are the only thing that can help?

Do they really believe that God created a flawed fertility system, then left generations of women to suffer before giving his blessing of medication? Or do they believe God has no authority over what happens in the labor room?

When faced with such beliefs, a Christian woman should remind herself that God created her body, and made her female. God designed the reproductive system and has been involved in the pregnancy since the conception. Then she should politely get up and leave. Yes, leave. Would you remain in the waiting room if your caregiver had a sign up that said, "I don't believe in God and neither should you." Then why would you remain in a childbirth class when the nurse tells you God has no desire to help you, and even if he did, he has no power?

In the Bible God tells us he is not only there, but he is in control of the labor and the birth!

> "Do I bring to the moment of birth and not give delivery?" says the Lord.
> "Do I close up the womb when I bring to delivery?" says your God. Isaiah 66:9

Technology is a gift from God, but only when it is used as a tool. A woman must do her best to educate herself, because there are risks to every technological intervention available. When it comes down to making a decision, she should face it prayerfully, asking God for wisdom as she weighs the risks and the benefits of each procedure.

What are some false teachings about labor that you have believed?

What is the truth about labor and birth, according to the Bible?

There is a flip side to our story. There is a segment of our population that has rejected the false teachings of the "need" for medication. Although they believe the female body is adequate to give birth, these teachers do not acknowledge God as the creator. Although they believe there is power for birth, they do not believe God is its source. Although they know birth is a spiritual event, it is not the Holy Spirit that they invite to be with them at this time.

I'm sure you have seen such teachers and learned about such classes. Perhaps you have even run away at the blatant paganism of such teachings. These new age philosophies tell women to use their own power, or to use the power of nature. They encourage the use of charms and chants, and meditation on some "spiritual" thing. They believe the atmosphere determines the "spirit" of the birth, rather than the Spirit controlling the atmosphere. They may be supporters of birth the way God created it, but they certainly have no interest in the one true God. In some instances, they may even suggest prayer to a false god. Once again the Christian should be reminded:

> *They exchanged the truth of God for a lie, and worshiped and served created things rather than the Creator—who is forever praised. Amen. Romans 1:25*

What evidence have you seen of such idol worship in your pregnancy and labor books?

What does the Bible say about serving false gods (idolatry)?

So what is a Christian woman to do? On one side being told God does not care and is powerless, on the other that he does not exist. Birth can be difficult enough without having to deal with people trying to make you give up your God. No wonder Christian women get fed up and give up on their desire for a normal yet spiritual birth.

Is it all coincidence that one of the most difficult things a woman will ever have to do is now controlled by people who tell her God can not or will not help. I doubt it. Satan knows when we are most tempted to turn to idols, and he is more than happy to encourage us to do just that.

In what ways have you personally experienced the spiritual battleground surrounding pregnancy and labor?

It is possible to give birth naturally, relying on God and not worshiping idols. It is also possible to choose to use medications or interventions and be relying on God. But it takes great discipline and a lot of work. The first thing you must do is pray, pray, pray. Let God know that you want to have him at your baby's birth. Ask him to open your eyes to false teaching and send you a teacher who will help you learn without attacking your God. Ask God to overcome your fears, and to strengthen your body for the upcoming birth. Ask God to protect you and your baby.

Then you must do what you can to educate yourself through books, magazines, and a good class in natural childbirth. You will know what you are learning is accurate if it gives both benefits and risks, and does not contradict the power or existence of God. Also, you must find a caregiver who respects your desire to depend on God, and use the technology only if necessary (i.e. emergency; many caregivers use technology so routinely, and rely on it so heavily that they may not be able to discern what is not necessary). This may involve changing caregivers, but in such cases you will be better off if you do.

Finally, you must work on the qualities we discussed in chapter 4 that are listed in 1 Timothy 2:15 *But women will be saved through childbearing-- if they continue in faith, love and holiness with propriety.* For this is what God told us we would need to be "saved" from the pains of childbirth. With these qualities developed, our bodies will be doing the same process, and the pain will be there, but the strength of the Lord will bring us through.

How do you know you are prepared to face the spiritual challenges ahead?

As you finish your time with God today, skim through the book up to this point, reading the verses given about birth. Do you recognize the power and authority God has over the act of giving birth? Sit at God's feet and have a "heart to heart" about your plans for your birth. Ask God what he thinks of your plans and tell him you are willing to submit your plan to his plan.

A Personal Discipline:

As you discuss your birth with the people in your life, listen carefully to their attitudes as they comment on the process of birth. When you are alone, record their comments (and yours) in your notebook and try to determine what belief (God does not exist, God is powerless or God is in control) the comment most supports. As you recognize comments that do not support the existence and power of God, train yourself to no longer say or believe them.

Chapter Six

Faith

You believe that there is one God. Good!
Even the demons believe that-and shudder. James 2:19

Every part of life has challenges that we must face, pregnancy and giving birth are no different. During this time you can choose to have faith in God, or you can choose not to trust God. In the most basic terms, it may seem that a "natural" birth is demonstrating faith while a medicated birth shows a lack of faith. However, you cannot define your faith by what happens to you in labor. That is backwards. Your faith should define how you respond to labor.

Let us begin by considering what faith is. Hebrews 11:1 tells us "Now faith is being sure of what we hope for and certain of what we do not see." Read the following passages and write down what you learn about faith from each of them.

Mark 5:22-34

James 2:14-24

If you have faith in God, you will do what he commands. You will do this because you trust that if you follow his commands, God will deal with you in the way he claimed he would. You trust that God will honor his end of the deal. Faith begins where just believing ends. But if you do not act on it, it is not faith. If you are truly living a life of faith, you should see evidence of serving God in your daily life. Read the following verses and write down what you learn about your faith from them.

Matthew 7:16-20

If your "fruit" does not give evidence of a good tree, take heart. The only difference between belief and faith is that faith is belief put into action. All you have to do is start living according to the promises of God through Jesus.

Knowing what faith is, we can turn our attention to how faith affects labor. For many women, the time of pregnancy prepares them for birth with fear, anxiety and worry. It seems there are no stories of normal pregnancies, and births. Instead women are reminded again and again about the small percentage of labors that are abnormal or dangerous. In some areas, it almost seems as if women compete to have the worst, most dangerous labor story to tell.

How can hearing stories of problems rather than stories of normal labors cause problems for women trying to build faith in God for labor?

The fear that can easily be instilled in a pregnant woman is going to affect her labor in a variety of ways. The most obvious way is that the body is designed to respond in specific ways to fear. Part of that response is to slow down or stop the labor process. While this may be useful if you are in a dangerous situation and need to get to safety, it isn't always helpful. For example, when laboring in a hospital a woman whose labor slows down will be treated as if it is a physical problem, not an emotional one, so she will receive interventions that are designed to speed up labor.

Another problem with fear is that it takes your energy and mental focus without giving you anything in return. Worry doesn't help a situation, it doesn't improve a situation, it only takes your emotional and mental energy away from productive tasks. This also works to separate you from God. When you worry, it becomes a constant battle to keep your eyes on God and your faith active to prevent fear from pulling you away from God's comfort. Don't think this is by accident. The time of pregnancy and giving birth are very spiritually fertile times, and fear is a weapon of spiritual warfare.

In what ways have you seen fear pull you away from God, not just in relation to this pregnancy, but in your whole life?

What fears during pregnancy and labor attack your faith in God?

Take a few minutes to read Hebrews Chapter 11, the chapter about faith. After you have read it, read the following verses and write their meaning in relation to your pregnancy and labor in your own words.

Romans 8:15

Philippians 4:6

Using faith in labor is not a formula. There is not a particular prayer or a comfort measure that you should do that shows you are laboring with faith. There is no one size fits all way to handle labor by faith, just as there is no one size fits all way to handle life by faith.

> *One man considers one day more sacred than another; another man considers every day alike. Each one should be fully convinced in his own mind. He who regards one day as special, does so to the Lord. He who eats meat, eats to the Lord, for he gives thanks to God; and he who abstains, does so to the Lord and gives thanks to God. For none of us lives to himself alone and none of us dies to himself alone. If we live, we live to the Lord; and if we die, we die to the Lord. So, whether we live or die, we belong to the Lord. Romans 14:5-8*

There is a fine line we draw here. On the one hand, you should not go into a normal labor planning an epidural because by doing so you demonstrate a lack of faith in God to help you handle any pain. But on the other hand, you cannot allow your baby to be harmed because accepting a medically necessary intervention would mean you didn't have faith. I wish there were some magic formula I could teach you to understand when to choose natural birth and when to choose medication. The best I can tell you is to educate yourself about normal birth and the options you have. That way you can make the best decision for the safety of you and your child if a situation arises during labor.

What are some ways a woman whose faith is in God during labor might handle contractions?

What are some ways a woman whose faith is in God during labor might handle problems in labor?

It is important to remember what faith is not. First, faith is not a substitute for an experienced doctor or midwife. Although faith may lead you to forgo certain tests and procedures, faith should not cause you to become haughty or proud to the point that you will not accept professional help in monitoring the progress of your pregnancy or birth. Even as far back as slavery in Egypt, midwives assisted pregnant women in ensuring health and monitoring the birth. However, the extent to which you seek assistance will depend on how much you need.

Your midwife is like a lifeguard, a watchman trained in birth to recognize when you need help and offer guidance and advice. She cannot make decisions for you, but she can assist you in finding information and by recommending ways for you to stay healthy. You hire her to serve your needs. Yet at the same time, faith is not signing away all responsibility for what happens to your doctor or midwife. It is still your right and responsibility to do what you need to do to stay healthy.

Faith is also not an excuse to do nothing when a problem arises. Rather than deal with hard issues, some women will claim they are trusting in God to solve the problem. Remember, faith is your belief in action, not reality in denial. Problems do arise in labor. But it is our faith that will allow us to work through our problems and grow closer to God at the same time.

Sometimes, even with great faith, God will not simply remove a problem. Paul asked repeatedly to be delivered of the thorn in his side, but God said "My grace is sufficient." If faith were a cure-all for every problem in life, surely Paul's thorn would have been taken away.

Sometimes, God does not desire a problem, but one is caused as a consequence to the decision or action of another person. God can remove the consequences, but frequently he does not. If you are hit by a car as you cross the street, God could heal your wounds instantly and have you back on your way. However it is more common that God allows the consequences to continue, and then he uses the problem that was created to draw you closer to Him.

Has God ever used a problem to draw you closer to him? How did it happen?

In the Bible there were women who died in childbirth, infants who died and there were women and children who were murdered. Bad things did happen. But bad things should not cause us to lose faith in God. God can do, and still does miracles. But the lack of a miraculous healing should not cause us to believe God is powerless.

If you do have a problem with your pregnancy or labor, it is no comfort when you realize you may never know how God used that problem to work for good. But God can be your comfort when you turn to him as your source of strength and support. Lean on him and cry on his shoulder. He will never grow weary of comforting you. Sometimes, all we may learn is to trust in God and to have fellowship with him during suffering.

Remember, you do not get to choose the circumstances of your labor. But you do get to choose how you respond to the circumstances.

A Personal Discipline

If you have not already, begin looking at the options that you have for labor and giving birth. Begin to work on your birth plan, considering each option not just for its ability to bring comfort or its impact on your health, but also about your faith and how your faith may affect its use.

Chapter Seven

Love

Think with me a moment about love. What does this word mean? How does it pertain to your birth? Why would Paul tell Timothy that Love was important to a woman's birth? Let's begin at the beginning. Look at these sentences:

I love you.
Love your neighbor.
Love the Lord your God.
For God so loved the world.

The first step in understanding love is to understand that love goes far beyond simply feeling a certain way about someone. God did not command us to feel lovingly towards others, although there are places where that is beneficial and desired. Instead, God commanded us to act in love by putting the needs of others before our own.

Dear children, let us not love with words or tongue but with actions and in truth. 1 John 3:18

In this same way, husbands ought to love their wives as their own bodies. He who loves his wife loves himself. After all, no one ever hated his own body, but he feeds and cares for it, just as Christ does the church. Ephesians 5:28- 29

What are some of the actions Paul considers to be a part of loving someone?

Taking care of someone's physical needs is part of loving them. This is why mothers are seen as such loving individuals, even if they are tired and frustrated, they feed their children, they change their child's diapers and in other ways ensure their child is cared for.

Yet love goes deeper than just meeting others physical needs. Love is the sacrificing of you for another.

> *This is how we know what love is: Jesus Christ laid down his life for us. And we ought to lay down our lives for our brothers. 1 John 3:16*
>
> *But God demonstrates his own love for us in this: While we were still sinners, Christ died for us. Romans 5:8*

Christ literally gave up his life. It is rare that we are called to die for another. Instead, we are called to give up our dreams, our goals, our desires, our wants and even our needs to fulfill the needs of others.

In what ways might you be called to lay down your life during pregnancy?

In what ways might you be called to lay down your life during labor?

To love your child, you will need to look out for his best interests. You may need to forgo certain habits during pregnancy to be sure he is as healthy as possible. If your pregnancy gets difficult, you may need to give up income to allow yourself more time to rest. You will need to allow your child space in your body, and to affect your body's functioning so he can grow and be healthy.

When labor comes, you will have the ultimate question laid before you, "Will you seek the good of your child over your comfort?"

No one will ask the question quite that way. A caregiver may ask if you would like "a little something" for the pain, "just to relax you, so you can enjoy the labor." But you need to be aware that this question is not as simple as it seems.

You see, every medication you take has an effect on your baby. Every drug that your doctor or midwife could give you will change the labor and affect the way your baby can respond to labor. This is why when a woman is given medications during labor she must wear an electric fetal monitor throughout the whole labor. The risk to the baby is greatly increased, so the baby is monitored to catch it quickly if something should happen.

The side effects of medications vary in frequency and intensity. They may make your child sleepy, may decrease the amount of oxygen he can get, cause respiratory problems, and even send an otherwise healthy child into fetal distress. These are all things that you must keep in mind when you are offered "a little something to move things along."

How do you feel about medications in labor knowing that they can have a huge impact on your baby's health?

Not every baby has visible side effects from medication. Some women are able to use the medication without any problem for mother or baby. But that does not mean that the risk does not exist.

When you take what is an ordinary, healthy and normal labor and introduce a medication to change labor (speed it up, remove the pain) you put risks on the baby that did not exist before. According to Henci Goer, the labor without medication has about a 5% chance of complication. Of those complications 75% fall into two very easily treatable categories – baby doesn't breathe right away or mother doesn't stop bleeding right away after the baby is born. Both of these are so easily treated that they can be taken care of in your home with portable equipment!

But we live in a society with a 25% cesarean section rate. Why is the rate so high if there only exists a 5% chance of a complication? The rate is high because the risks are increased with every intervention performed. The rates for pain and labor stimulating medications are overwhelming. Increasing the risk during labor does cause problems.

> *Be on your guard; stand firm in the faith; be men of courage; be strong. Do everything in love. 1 Corinthians 16:13,14*

The commands of God do not change because you are in labor. The requirements of God are not lessened because you are going through a difficult trial. Rather, it is through trials that our faith is tested. You will be tested in labor. You must remain faithful to God, and serve your baby in love. You must make decisions based on what is healthiest and the lowest risk for your child. In 95% of cases, this will be a labor without medication.

What is your initial response to the previous paragraph?

Stop here and pray. Come back to the study in an hour or two, or in a few days if necessary, when you have wrestled with these statements and have poured your heart out to God.

How has your response to the above paragraph changed?

The season of life in which you are pregnant, give birth and care for a newborn is not only a time of tremendous growth for your baby, it is an incredible time of spiritual growth for you. I firmly believe that God has designed it that way. While pregnant a woman's mind travels to her spiritual condition – what kind of mother will she be, how will she teach her children to love God, how will she help her children not make the same mistakes she has made. This openness to the Holy Spirit brings about growth at a phenomenal rate.

The spiritual growth during pregnancy and birth is a real danger to the enemy. He doesn't want mother's growing in faith and love, testing their spiritual muscles and finding out how strong God is. Doesn't it make sense that such a fertile time for personal growth would be a time that is attacked by fear? This fear allows the enemy to change our thoughts from our spiritual condition to dread of the upcoming labor. In effect, it gets our eyes off God and onto ourselves. When full-blown, this fear gets us to act in selfishness; putting our baby's health and well-being at risk in an attempt to prevent a time of discomfort and pain.

I am going to say this again, because it is important for you to understand that taking medications during a normal labor increases the risks for you and your baby. Taking medications when there is no medical emergency or true cause for medications puts your baby at risk unnecessarily. You are choosing your comfort over your baby's health. This cannot be made light of for a Christian who is called to love others sacrificially.

God is gracious, and he does give you free will. He does not remove the option of using medications during labor from you. He does not force you to labor without pain relieving medication. However, do not forget his call to you. Do not use your freedom to sin.

> You, my brothers, were called to be free. But do not use your freedom to indulge the sinful nature; rather, serve one another in love. The entire law is summed up in a single command: "Love your neighbor as yourself."
> Galatians 5:13-14

God has given you the ability and the strength to do what is right. The Bible tells us that every time we are tempted, God helps us to stand up under it. I urge you not to look forward to the work of labor with fear, but understanding the power you have in Christ Jesus.

> For God did not give us a spirit of timidity, but a spirit of power, of love and of self-discipline. 2 Timothy 1:7

In what ways are you approaching labor with timidity?

In what ways are you approaching labor with power, love and self-discipline?

As a doula, I have been trained that a woman always has the right to choose to use medication during labor. I have never tried to talk a woman out of using medication when she asked in labor because I firmly believe that it is not a decision that I can make for her. God used a friend of mine just this morning to tell me that I have been trained wrong.

My sweet friend, with a beautiful heart, was kindly telling an expectant mother that she has always found that she needed someone to hold her accountable to doing what is right when she is struggling with difficult things. She said, "So, I asked my husband to keep me accountable to not using medication unless there was a medical problem, and he did." This friend was more ready than I had been for the rigors of labor. By asking someone to keep her accountable she was strengthening the commitment she had made to act in her baby's best interest.

Please understand that accountability is not the same as deciding for you. Accountability is only holding you accountable to what you said you would do. Reminding you of decisions you had made and helping you to follow those decisions. It is not forcing you to follow decisions. In labor, you may ask someone to remind you that you had wanted to labor a particular way and if you change you mind to ask you a question such as, "Do you think this is the best thing for the baby right now?"

Who will keep you accountable to love during labor?

Two important points must be made here. First, there may come a time in a small percentage of labors at which the risk of not using a medication or an intervention outweighs the risk of using the medication. If this happens, it is more loving to accept the intervention which reduces the risk than to not accept an intervention. For some women, this will be a struggle because they had their heart set on a particular style or type of labor which will no longer be available, and yes, using an intervention can be and often is a loving sacrifice for your child when this happens. Remember, the point of loving is putting the needs of someone else ahead of your own. That can just as easily mean accepting an intervention when you wanted a natural birth as it can mean having a natural birth when you would have preferred medication.

The second point is that it is not enough to decide to labor without medication to love your child, you must learn how to labor and your assistants must learn how to help you. If you have never been through labor before, you may be surprised at how unfamiliar your body is to the work that needs to be done. It can take tremendous effort to work through the contractions, to step aside and let your body work. You need to prepare by learning different techniques to work with your body instead of against it.

Unless you understand the difference between normal and complication, you will not be able to discern when the risk to your baby is increased or decreased by the use of medication. You need to understand what is normal in labor. You also need to know what options are available if a complication arises. You may be surprised to learn that there are medical and non-medical ways to handle many of the common variations of labor. In general, it is best to use the non-medical methods first since they generally involve the least amount of risk for the baby.

In order for a childbirth attendant, husband or coach to be helpful to you in labor, you BOTH need to understand the best ways to handle labor. You need to be familiar with the normal labor process and several coping strategies. Asking a woman to labor without medication without giving her the tools and knowledge she needs to labor effectively is like asking someone to swim without a life-jacket when they have never been in the water before. "*Carry each other's burdens, and in this way you will fulfill the law of Christ.*" (Galatians 6:2). A labor coach should work with the woman to help her find the positions, techniques and comfort measures that help her stay as comfortable as possible during labor. A coach who refuses to allow you to use medication without helping you handle contractions is cruel.

What do you need to do before labor to be able to love your baby sacrificially?

A Personal Discipline

This week, make a point of sending "love notes" to your baby. When you make a decision to put your baby's health above your comfort (such as when you choose to drink milk or water rather than soda; or when you decide to go for a walk after dinner to help indigestion instead of grabbing the Tums) put it on a piece of paper and stick it someplace where you will see it throughout the week. Thank God for helping you learn how to love.

Chapter Eight

Holiness

Does the idea of being "holy" seem too unreal? After all, you are just a sinner. How can you be holy?   The word from 1 Timothy 2:15 that was translated to mean holiness, can also mean purity. Because it can be easier to understand the word pure, we will substitute it here for the discussion.

Unfortunately "pure" is an old-fashioned word.   Does it conjure up images of plainly dressed young women without makeup and unattractive hair?   If so, you need a different definition of pure!

When God tells us to be pure, he is not directing us to be boring, but to be pure in heart.   That means that your heart belongs to God 100%. Think of it like a garden. If you were to seed a bed of daisies, but when the seed grew it was 75% daisies and 25% petunias you would say the seed was not pure. The seed must have been mixed up, because if it were pure you would have 100% daisies.

It is the same way with the garden in your heart. When you look at what is planted, does it glorify God? Or is your heart garden speckled or even peppered with weeds? If there are weeds in your heart garden, then you know the seed you have been using is not pure. In other words, there must be portions of your life that you have not given to God to control.

Guessing, what percentage of your heart do you think is under God's control?

Who or what controls the other parts of your heart?

One of the dangers of being a Christian is that we begin to judge others, and compare ourselves to them. As we are more and more aware of how far we have come from the sins we used to do, we begin to feel good, worthy and possibly even that we have "made it." After all, you've come so much farther than the other people. Why, if they had learned even half of what you did, they would not be still sinning.

Oh, if I could only warn you about the danger of this type of prideful thinking. If you are even toying with the idea that you have "made it" and can take a "day off from God" here and there you have devoted your life to very impure seed. Paul himself complained more and more of his sinfulness as he grew closer and closer to God. It is impossible to be building a relationship with God while you are building up yourself.

Let me put that another way. God is the most perfect being in the universe. He is all powerful, all knowing, all seeing, sinless, creative and God is love. The closer you get to God, the more you will recognize your own sinfulness. So, rather than thinking higher of yourself (pride), you will begin to be humbled.

There are other impurities that can enter your heart besides pride, although pride is a common problem. Essentially, these impurities are idols, things we turn to other than God.

> *Put to death, therefore, whatever belongs to your earthly nature: sexual immorality, impurity, lust, evil desires and greed, which is idolatry. Colossians 3:5*

Why do you think greed is considered idolatry?

What are some other idols we make today?

Are you recognizing some idols that have been set up in your life? Are there things that you have trusted in when you should have trusted God? Read Psalm 51:10. Then stop right here and say a prayer similar to this Psalm, ask God to make your heart pure:

> *Create in me a pure heart, O God,*
> *and renew a steadfast spirit within me.*

How do you get a pure heart? Where does it come from? The Psalmist asked that same question, and also gave an answer.

> *How can a young man keep his way pure?*
> *By living according to your word. Psalm 119:9*

Write the meaning of Psalm 119:9 in your own words.

Review your life from the past month. Have you lived pure, devoted to God? Use this space to list instances you would like to bring before God, and be sure to ask his help in changing the way you handle future situations.

Are you not sure if you have lived a pure life? There may be several reasons for your uncertainty. You can not live according to God's Word if you don't know what his Word says. When you are caught in a trial and look at your WWJD bracelet, do you even know what Jesus would have done? It can be interesting sometimes to make suppositions and discuss philosophy, but you can not substitute your thoughts on what God might be like for God's Word which tells you exactly what God is like.

I am jealous for you with a godly jealousy. I promised you to one husband, to Christ, so that I might present you as a pure virgin to him. But I am afraid that just as Eve was deceived by the serpent's cunning, your minds may somehow be led astray from your sincere and pure devotion to Christ. For if someone comes to you and preaches a Jesus other than the Jesus we preached, or if you receive a different spirit from the one you received, or a different gospel from the one you accepted, you put up with it easily enough. 2 Corinthians 11:2-4

If you are not regularly in God's Word (reading the Bible) you become susceptible to false teachings that sound good to your ears, but contradict what God says.

The goal of this command is love, which comes from a pure heart and a good conscience and a sincere faith. Some have wandered away from these and turned to meaningless talk. They want to be teachers of the law, but they do not know what they are talking about or what they so confidently affirm.
1 Timothy 1:5-7

For the time will come when men will not put up with sound doctrine. Instead, to suit their own desires, they will gather around them a great number of teachers to say what their itching ears want to hear. They will turn their ears away from the truth and turn aside to myths. 2 Timothy 4:3-4

Here is another test. When faced with a problem, do you turn to the latest psychological research to see how you should act, or do you turn to God's Word. It is sad when Christians put more faith in the latest survey then the wisdom of the Almighty God. Sure, there is a lot of new information about health, interpersonal relationships and romance everyday.   But not every piece of advice can stand up to the test of God's Word. When faced with choosing God's Word over man's wisdom, which do you pick?

Satan has encouraged us to think in terms of stark black and white, good and bad so that we become confused in the gray areas. We look at the shades of gray and say, "but is surely isn't black, so it must be ok." But goodness was never meant to be judged according to evil. Goodness must be measured by the standard of God. Any shade of gray will look bright and light when placed next to black. But when you put in next to a pure white, you see how really dark it is. We need to retrain ourselves to say, "this isn't white, so it must be bad."

> But mark this: There will be terrible times in the last days. People will be lovers of themselves, lovers of money, boastful, proud, abusive, disobedient to their parents, ungrateful, unholy, without love, unforgiving, slanderous, without self-control, brutal, not lovers of the good, treacherous, rash, conceited, lovers of pleasure rather than lovers of God—having a form of godliness but denying its power. Have nothing to do with them. 2 Timothy3: 1-5

Understanding now the danger of shades of gray, why would Paul tell us to have nothing to do with the types of people listed in 2 Timothy 3:1-5

But the question is, what does purity (or holiness) have to do with having a baby? Purity is important during labor because you cannot suddenly start calling on God during labor when you are exhausted and stripped of the mask you wear every day. This mask is a filter for your thoughts, only letting you do or say the things that are socially appropriate.   Many people allow themselves to entertain thoughts and ideas that they would never speak or do. If you only appear to serve God, but secretly serve an idol, you will serve your idol during labor.   Labor takes so much energy you cannot afford to keep your mask on while you labor. Your true heart will show. If you want to call on God during labor you need to have a heart that calls on him naturally.

Take a look at your life this past month. What percentage of your life was spent serving and worshiping God, and what part was spent serving and worshiping your caregiver, your pregnancy, your desire for a specific type of labor, your joy at becoming a mother? Did you trust in God 90% and your caregiver 10%? Even worshiping your caregiver only 1% is not being pure. Do not mistake the minister for the God he serves! Did you celebrate God for sending you blessings, or did you worship the creation rather than the creator?

Have you been expecting to labor on your strength rather than on the strength of God? Have you been planning for a specific labor as if the goal were to labor a special way rather than to love and serve God? Did your prayers stop because you finally got pregnant, so you didn't need to ask God to make you pregnant any longer? Remember, pregnancy and childbearing are spiritually fertile times in your life. To be sure that you are growing in the right direction, you need to keep your eyes focused on God. Purity is important for your growth and maturity.

As you end your time with God today, ask him to tear away from you the idols you have been serving. God wants your heart to be pure. In fact, God tells us to be holy, because he is holy. Do not think that you cannot give up your idols. They have no hold on you. God is bigger than any idol you are serving. God not only has the power to defeat your idol, but he also has the desire. Remember, God will be working with you when you ask him to make your heart pure.

A Personal Discipline

This week, as you begin to recognize the idols that you serve, make a list in your notebook. At the end of each day, confess to God your impure heart and ask him to help you destroy your idol. You may find it helpful to write the name of your idol on a paper, and then throw out or destroy the paper.

Chapter Nine

Propriety

Strong's Greek Dictionary defines propriety as soundness of mind or self-control. To learn how this fits in with birth, we must study what the Bible has to say about self-control. Read each of the following passages. In the space provided, write what God teaches you about self-control from each set of verses.

> *Be self-controlled and alert. Your enemy the devil prowls around like a roaring lion looking for someone to devour. Resist him, standing firm in the faith, because you know that your brothers throughout the world are undergoing the same kind of sufferings. 1 Peter 5:8-9*

> *For this very reason, make every effort to add to your faith goodness; and to goodness, knowledge; 6and to knowledge, self-control; and to self-control, perseverance; and to perseverance, godliness; and to godliness, brotherly kindness; and to brotherly kindness, love. For if you possess these qualities in increasing measure, they will keep you from being ineffective and unproductive in your knowledge of our Lord Jesus Christ. 2 Peter 1:5-8*

Like a city whose walls are broken down is a man who lacks self-control. Proverbs 25:28

It becomes clear that self-control is a matter of extreme importance for leading a godly life. In fact, self-control is our "wall of protection" against the temptations of Satan. Without self-control, we give in to any scheme, plan or lie that is thrown at us.

Think of your body as having two parts. There is the physical body and the spiritual body. The physical body, which is composed of blood and tissues, is constantly bombarded by signals from the world around you. Your hands, eyes, mouth; your whole physical body is constantly discerning whether it is in pleasure or pain. If it were left up to your physical body, it would constantly be seeking more and better pleasure, which is the greatest desire of the physical body.

Your spiritual body is discerning. It takes the information that the physical body receives and uses it to determine whether or not the action desired by your physical body is in line with God's will. Your spiritual body is constantly determining which desired actions are outside of God's will. The nature of your spiritual body is such that it is not able to override the actions of the physical body without the physical body using self-control. That means that your physical body must deny itself some of its desires to remain in line with God's will.

Read these verses that describe the importance of self-control. In the space provided, write in your own words how that verse tells you to use self-control to prevent sin.

For the grace of God that brings salvation has appeared to all men. It teaches us to say "No" to ungodliness and worldly passions, and to live self-controlled, upright and godly lives in this present age, while we wait for the blessed hope—the glorious appearing of our great God and Savior, Jesus Christ, who gave himself for us to redeem us from all wickedness and to purify for himself a people that are his very own, eager to do what is good. Titus 2:11-14

Therefore, prepare your minds for action; be self-controlled; set your hope fully on the grace to be given you when Jesus Christ is revealed. As obedient children, do not conform to the evil desires you had when you lived in ignorance. But just as he who called you is holy, so be holy in all you do; for it is written: "Be holy, because I am holy." 1 Peter 1:13-16

It is no secret that we live in a society that does not consider self-control as a quality worth seeking. We are constantly bombarded by the message that we should satisfy ourselves when we want with whatever will please us. Stop for a moment and try to recall the last commercial or advertisement that you saw. What were they selling, and what was the message they used to sell that product to you?

No matter what the product, I am sure the message was along the lines of "you can have more, (or do more, or be more, or feel more) with this product." We are sold on self-indulgence. We have bought into the marketing scheme and become dissatisfied with our lives. We are convinced that the only way to find happiness (or comfort, or health, or beauty, or love) is to buy just one more thing, eat just one more dessert, try just one more miracle cure face lotion.

Why do we allow ourselves to fall for these lies? If we ever stopped to think, we would realize they are lies before we bought that coffee maker that was going to make breakfast the most romantic meal of the day and become our reason to get out of bed in the morning! Look around you. How many lies have you believed? How many times did you try to improve your life with one of these worthless products? We lack self-control.

But we are not just indulging in our greed for stuff and our greed for food. We are also indulging in our lusts. Unless you are the rare woman, you have probably watched a television show or movie that contained questionable or outright sinful behaviors. Why do we put up with wasting our time enjoying other people's sins? The desire to watch others engaged in sexual encounters used to make you a voyeur, now it makes you a movie fan. We can make all the excuses we want, but the bottom line is still, we lack self-control.

Self-control must be developed. Its very nature goes against the desires of your physical body, and so seems unpleasant. But you must discipline yourself to use self-control when your spiritual body tells you not to do something. This is very difficult at first, but will become easier with practice. Self-control is like a muscle, the more you use it, the stronger it gets.

In what areas of your life have you failed to develop self-control?

What was the lie(s) that you believed that encouraged you to indulge?

What is God's truth about that lie(s)?

If you don't know what God says about your specific sins, you need to start spending more time in your Bible. Use a concordance to find what the Bible has to say about the areas that interest you. God wants you to know the truth. If you ask, he will tell you.

Self-control is important for more reasons that keeping us from sin. It also helps to keep us from the consequences of sin. If you want to review the impact sin can have on your life, go back to the chapter on Holiness. As an example, have you had difficulty with your prayer life? Do you find it difficult to converse with God on a regular basis? Do you feel distant from God when you pray? Perhaps you need to develop some self-control.

*The end of all things is near. Therefore be clear minded
and self-controlled so that you can pray. 1 Peter 4:7*

Summarize what this verses means. How does it relate to Psalm 66:18, "If I had cherished sin in my heart, the Lord would not have listened."

Pregnancy can be a time of testing your self-control. You are expected to eat healthier, get regular exercise and stop any practices that may be unhealthy for your baby. Some women have trouble with heart-burn or indigestion but won't stop eating foods that make them sick, or eat smaller meals to prevent the stomach overload. These women lack the self-control to tell themselves "no" when they want to overeat.

Other women do not slow down their lives to be sure they get enough rest. These women lack the self-control to be content with doing less. On the other hand, some women unnecessarily slow down to a stop during pregnancy, these women lack the self-control to disciple their bodies to complete regular activities and exercise. Some women use pregnancy as an excuse to remove all self-control from their relationships. These women demand through screaming or whining that others bend over backward to meet their whims and desires.

Many women find that labor is a time of great trial and testing. Some women, although they know that God is able to be their source of comfort and strength, give up because they feel it is too difficult to go on. These women lack the self-control to restrain their bodies desire to end the difficult situation. They are unhappy with God's timing and decide to manage the labor themselves. Do not underestimate the importance of self-control on your ability to give birth naturally. You must be able to tell your body "No" when it wants to give up on God. You also need to have the self-control to let your body do the work it needs to do without fighting it.

As you end you time with God today, meditate on the following two verses. Consider the importance self-control has for your pregnancy and labor.

> *But the fruit of the Spirit is love, joy, peace, patience, kindness, goodness, faithfulness, gentleness and self-control. Against such things there is no law. Galatians 5:22-23*

> *For this very reason, make every effort to add to your faith goodness; and to goodness, knowledge; and to knowledge, self-control; and to self-control, perseverance; and to perseverance, godliness; and to godliness, brotherly kindness; and to brotherly kindness, love. For if you possess these qualities in increasing measure, they will keep you from being ineffective and unproductive in your knowledge of our Lord Jesus Christ. But if anyone does not have them, he is nearsighted and blind, and has forgotten that he has been cleansed from his past sins. 2 Peter 1:5-9*

A Personal Discipline

This week, work out your self-control muscle. Think of one or two sins that have been constant in your life. For one week, deny yourself the indulgence of this sin. If it is gossip, don't let yourself speak about other people.   If it is pornography, don't allow yourself to even glance at it. If it is greed, don't go to any store, not even the grocery store (I will bet your family can eat very well on the food you already have in the house, or someone else can go to the grocery store for you so you have no excuses). How difficult or easy was it to overcome that particular sin in each instance.   Do you see a trend of strengthening in your self-control?

Chapter Ten

Becoming a Mother

When Jesus was asked what the greatest command was, he answered that it was to love God. He said the second greatest was to love others. Your journey in motherhood will be a journey in learning how to love.

If you are nervous about having to love and care for someone 24 hours a day, please do not despair. There are two things you need to know. The first is that pregnancy prepares you perfectly to be a mother. The second is that God will meet your needs, so you can focus on the needs of your baby.

I cannot think of a more loving thing a person can do than to give their body for someone else. You have been doing this for several months now. You have dealt with the inconveniences of backaches, tiredness, nausea, sore breasts, frequent bathroom trips and whatever other "problem" your pregnancy has thrown at you. You may even have had a terrible illness during pregnancy, but you did not get rid of the baby.

Had you considered that before? Had you thought about how much you "suffered" for your child? Some women are very aware of how much they suffer, and let everyone know. They are the first to tell you how terrible their pregnancy and labors were. They have every kind of horror story you can imagine, and spare you no detail in telling them. Some go so far as to say it was so bad they would never do it again. I am not talking about that kind of an awareness of suffering.

In the part of Matthew known as the Sermon on the Mount, Jesus told the listeners

"When you fast, do not look somber as the hypocrites do, for they disfigure their faces to show men they are fasting. I tell you the truth, they have received their reward in full. But when you fast, put oil on your head and wash your face, so that it will not be obvious to men that you are fasting, but only to your Father, who is unseen; and your Father, who sees what is done in secret, will reward you. Matthew 6:16-18

Indulge me for a moment as I make some correlations between what Jesus teaches about fasting, and about our society's views of pregnancy.

First, notice that the "hypocrites" disfigure their faces while fasting. This is done presumably, so that everyone will know that they are fasting and will think more highly of them for their great sacrifice for God. But Jesus makes it clear that this kind of sacrifice is not done for God, but for men. The sacrifice God desires from fasting is done in secret, not for the praise of others but for the glory of God.

Second, notice that Jesus tells the crowd that putting on a performance of suffering for God only gives you the attention of men, but actually fasting for God will give you a reward from your Father in heaven.

Relating this to the suffering of pregnancy, think back to the woman who made it obvious that she was suffering. Every ache and pain is groaned at loudly to gain the attention of those surrounding her. She is not suffering for God, or for her baby, but is suffering for herself. She is complaining of the very things she hopes to feel because they give her attention. That is why Jesus refers to these people as hypocrites. But what of the woman who suffers the same inconveniences without complaint? This woman has just as many trips to the bathroom, but rather than moan and groan, she sings praises because it is a reminder of the way God has blessed her. It is a reminder that her baby is still with her.

Think also of the reward. All the complaining woman gets is the attention of her friends, co-workers and family. Perhaps she gets sympathy at the beginning of her pregnancy, but probably not for long. In the end she sees her baby as a way to get attention. To put it less delicately, she uses her baby to meet her own desires. She starts her life as a new mother having taught herself to resent her baby, and the most difficult times are yet to begin. But the non-complaining woman has already developed a deep love for her child by enduring the pregnancy. This woman is focused on meeting the needs of her baby, and is prepared to meet the challenges of mothering with patience and strength.

What are some specific rewards that God may give a woman who suffers for God and her baby rather than for the attention of others?

Do you find yourself complaining about being pregnant?

If so, what does this say about your desire to mother a child?

If you do complain about being pregnant, stop here and pray that God will change your heart to help you focus on the baby rather than the inconveniences.

What about a woman who has a real problem? What about a woman for whom pregnancy is a very difficult time, and every day is spent in wonder about the life of the baby? This may be hard to take, but the Bible does not give her permission to complain either. Yes, she does need to inform her caregivers about what is happening, but she does not need to complain to people who can do nothing about the situation.

There is a difference between complaining and seeking help. You can call a friend and ask her for help without complaining about things she cannot prevent or cure. There is a difference between seeking advice and complaining. There is a difference between updating loved ones and complaining.

Not complaining does not mean that you stop communicating with people, or that you don't share unpleasant or difficult news with them. But it does mean that you recognize that people can never fully meet your needs for comfort, solace, encouragement, love and support. Only God can fulfill you. Many times women will complain about what they cannot change rather than admit their frustration to God to allow him to start healing them.

Essentially, complaining says, "God, I don't think you are handling this situation right. I don't think you are making the right decisions." It comes from a heart of pride. The worst part is that a complaining heart is never satisfied. You will always find something you do not agree with. But you have to have faith that God is still in control, and that his decisions will work for good.

If you are unsure of this, read the book of Job. In his story, Job lost all his possessions, his family and his health. Yet Job would not allow himself to complain because he understood that God was in control. Job did feel bold enough to ask God why he did it, but God never gave him an answer. He simply stated that he was God, and that was enough.

How are you handling the discomforts of pregnancy?

How does it show you trust that God is in control?

How do the inconveniences of pregnancy prepare you to be a mother? In God's infinite wisdom, he designed pregnancy to be a time of strengthening your mothering skills by practicing them every day. What are these skills? The list is very long, but to get you started, here are some of the things you learn while pregnant.

Trusting God
Receiving subtle cues from your baby
Patience
Perseverance
Ability to wake several times at night
Being joyful through difficulties

God has designed this time of pregnancy to prepare you by developing all the skills you will need to be a Godly mother. The most important of these skills is to trust God. If you do not trust God, your mothering will feel more like carrying the weight of the world.

Why is trust in God so important? Because during the first few weeks of your baby's life, you will feel helpless, confused and frustrated. You will no longer be able to lean on yourself the way you had in your pre-baby days. You will not have the strength to do it alone. You must simply release control of your situation to God, he is a much better organizer anyway.

Trusting in God will free you to meet the needs of your new baby. If you don't trust God will refresh you, even with "enough" sleep, you will become frustrated and possibly angry at your child for taking away what you consider to be your rights. If you don't trust that God is able to arrange to have the housework done, you may place your new baby in a swing or chair alone for many hours each day while you concentrate on the less important things. God will provide for your needs. Let him bless you, so you can spend your time blessing your baby.

In my experience, no amount of discussion can prepare a woman for the changes she undergoes in the first few weeks after the baby is born. For that reason I will stop my discussion here and simply give you a list of verses that you can use to overcome the frustrations that await you.

For Lack of Sleep

Psalm 63:6-9
On my bed I remember you;
I think of you through the watches of the night.
Because you are my help,
I sing in the shadow of your wings.
My soul clings to you;
your right hand upholds me.

Psalm 119:148
My eyes stay open through the watches of the night,
that I may meditate on your promises.

Psalm 121:3-4
He will not let your foot slip—
he who watches over you will not slumber;
indeed, he who watches over Israel
will neither slumber nor sleep.

Psalm 143:8
Let the morning bring me word of your unfailing love,
for I have put my trust in you.
Show me the way I should go,
for to you I lift up my soul.

Lamentations 2:19
Arise, cry out in the night,
as the watches of the night begin;
pour out your heart like water
in the presence of the Lord.
Lift up your hands to him
for the lives of your children,
who faint from hunger
at the head of every street

When You are Overcome by Mealtimes

1 Corinthians 10:31
So whether you eat or drink or whatever you do,
do it all for the glory of God.

John 6:27
Do not work for food that spoils, but for food that
endures to eternal life, which the Son of Man will give
you. On him God the Father has placed his seal of
approval."

1 Corinthians 8:8
But food does not bring us near to God;
we are no worse if we do not eat, and no better if we do.

Concerning Your Attitude

1 Corinthians 4:21
What do you prefer? Shall I come to you with a whip,
or in love and with a gentle spirit?

Hebrews 12:11
No discipline seems pleasant at the time, but painful.
Later on, however, it produces a harvest of
righteousness and peace for those who have been
trained by it.

Hebrews 13: 15-16
Through Jesus, therefore, let us continually offer to God
a sacrifice of praise—the fruit of lips that confess his
name. And do not forget to do good and to share with
others, for with such sacrifices God is pleased.

1 Thessalonians 5:16-18
Be joyful always; pray continually; give thanks in all
circumstances, for this is God's will for you in Christ
Jesus.

When You Are Not Sure You Can Handle
Being Someone's Mom

2 Corinthians 3:4-6
Such confidence as this is ours through Christ before God. Not that we are competent in ourselves to claim anything for ourselves, but our competence comes from God. He has made us competent as ministers of a new covenant—not of the letter but of the Spirit; for the letter kills, but the Spirit gives life.

2 Samuel 22:33
It is God who arms me with strength and makes my way perfect.

James 1:5-6
If any of you lacks wisdom, he should ask God, who gives generously to all without finding fault, and it will be given to him. But when he asks, he must believe and not doubt, because he who doubts is like a wave of the sea, blown and tossed by the wind. That man should not think he will receive anything from the Lord; he is a double-minded man, unstable in all he does.

Psalm 25:16
Turn to me and be gracious to me, for I am lonely and afflicted.

Psalm 42:5
Why are you downcast, O my soul? Why so disturbed within me? Put your hope in God, for I will yet praise him, my Savior and my God.

Psalm 34:17-18
The righteous cry out, and the Lord hears them; he delivers them from all their troubles. The Lord is close to the brokenhearted and saves those who are crushed in spirit.

Making Difficult Decisions

Ephesians 5:15-16

Be very careful, then, how you live—not as unwise but as wise, making the most of every opportunity, because the days are evil.

Romans 8:28-29

And we know that in all things God works for the good of those who love him, who have been called according to his purpose.

Psalm 27:1

*The Lord is my light and my salvation—
whom shall I fear?
The Lord is the stronghold of my life—
of whom shall I be afraid?*

About the Author

Jennifer Vanderlaan is a childbirth educator and doula living in upstate New York. She created the Birthing Naturally website, co-founded the Cascade Christian Childbirth Association and developed a local volunteer doula ministry. She received degrees in physiology and psychology from Michigan State University, studied through The Academy of Husband Coached Childbirth®, Doulas of North America and trained childbirth educators through the Childbirth and Postpartum Professional 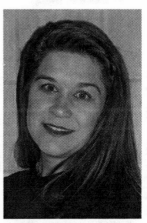 Association. Her materials are used in childbirth classes around the country.

Jennifer married her husband, Jeff, in 1995. They moved from Michigan to New York so Jeff could serve as minister to the students at The University at Albany. They have been blessed with two children, Josette and Jaron. They have experienced two normal, natural births; one at home and one in a hospital.

Jennifer explains that she writes out of her desire to share what she has learned with other women. Much of the material for The Lord of Birth comes straight from her personal prayer journals she kept during each of her pregnancies. For more of Jennifer's writings about pregnancy and childbirth, please visit her website where you will find information about staying healthy, preparing for labor and natural childbirth comfort measures.

www.birthingnaturally.net

CASCADE CHRISTIAN CHILDBIRTH

www.christianchildbirth.org